Live Well & Love Yourself:

A Reflective Guide to Living a Life with Passion and Purpose

Lauren Kissee

Copyright © 2018 Lauren Kissee

All rights reserved.

ISBN: 9781792798894

CONTENTS

Foreward

1	Where I Came From	1
2	Who You are is Enough	9
3	Who Do You Need to Forgive?	15
4	What Make You Come Alive?	21
5	Learn to Say No (The Joy Test)	27
6	Overcoming Insecurity	31
7	Self-Talk	37
8	Your Healthiest Self is Your Most Confident Self	43
9	Take the Road Less Travelled	55
10	Affirmations	59
	Closing	67
	Acknowledgements	71
	References	73

FOREWARD

    As a young child, I remember being acutely aware of how I looked in comparison to others. I have a vivid memory of being about 6 years old on a hot summer day in Southern California. My cousin and I were playing water games around the pool when I noticed that she looked different than me. Her belly was flat but as I looked down, I saw that mine was round. As a six-year-old, I didn't know why we looked different, but I didn't like it. At six years old, I didn't know the meaning of fat or skinny. All I knew was that I had a round buddha-belly and my cousin's belly was flat. That was my first memory of self-loathing.

    The journey to self-love is not an easy one. It's often hindered by comparison, disappointment, and self-loathing. I've read all the cute captions about self-love and I've done all of the things that I've been told boost confidence, but none of these have helped me.

Loving yourself isn't a box you check off the list. It isn't a certain milestone you hit in life. I've spent the last 25 years of my life learning to love who I was created to be and it's still a struggle some days. I'm not only talking about body image, either. Self-acceptance is so much more than that. This is my journey to self-love. This is my journey from a life of stress, self-criticism, and unrealistic expectations to a life of peace, contentment, and inner strength. This is what has worked on my journey and what hasn't. This is a journey about focusing more on where you're going than where you have been. This is a journey about grace & forgiveness.

You may be wondering, what the heck "self-love" is anyway? Dictionary.com defines it as, "regard for one's own well-being and happiness." I define self-love as being grateful and in love with your life. This means having genuine love for yourself and for your unique talents and abilities. Self-love does not mean living a life of selfishness. This book is the product of my personal conviction that loving yourself is truly the only way you will have the capacity to best love and serve others. This book isn't going to teach you to love yourself so that you put yourself on a pedestal or act better than anyone else. This book is going to show you how to genuinely appreciate and take care of yourself so that you are able to love others more deeply.

1 WHERE I CAME FROM

I am who I am because of the strong-willed women in my family. I love my family with all of my heart and I am extremely blessed to come from a family that has such strong values. I come from a family of achievers. As a young child, I remember being taught that productivity, accomplishment, and perfection was the standard. This upbringing taught me to excel at anything I put my mind to because I had a strong work-ethic and was determined to succeed. That being said, self-love was not something I was ever taught. I was taught that feelings aren't worth spending time on and that I'm not important enough to focus on myself. The word "selfish" was used often in my household whenever I expressed a personal desire. I quickly learned to do everything in my power to never be called selfish.

Even as a young child, I was taught that there is always more to do, more to stress about, and more to achieve. Schedules and to-do lists were a part of my life from a very early age and I quickly learned that the end of a to-do list is only the beginning of another one. There was no room to be average. I felt the pressure every day to be more than I already was.

In middle school, I remember wanting to wear makeup but being told that I shouldn't be focused on vanity. If I ever had an attitude, my family would worry that I would turn into a "problem child." Everything was so extreme in my childhood. I was unintentionally taught to be self-critical and even self-deprecating at times. As someone who loved performing, making up dance routines, and putting on a show, I always struggled with this inward feeling that something must be wrong with me. I must be too self-centered. I must not think about anyone other than myself. I must push aside my own wants and aspirations in order to have a successful life that is worthy of my family's approval.

My mother had my best intentions in mind and was raising me simply how she had been raised. I am so thankful that I was taught how to be disciplined, a self-starter, and a quick learner. I was pushed to work hard and excel in everything I do, and I am grateful for that. With every good lesson though, came a side of shame. Nothing I did was ever good enough. I learned to have unreachable expectations for myself. I never learned to love myself. I learned to love what I did, not who I was. I learned to chase accolades and accomplishments rather than grow into the person God had already created me to be.

Because I had the mindset that nothing I ever did would be

enough, I was very critical of myself and my body image. I have always strived for perfection and even though I was completely healthy & fit, it was never enough for me. Being critical of my body image didn't come from insecurity, but from my desire for perfection. At some point in high school, I just stopped caring. I realized that I would never obtain the perfect body, so I stopped caring about my health in general.

This led to a downward spiral of poor health. I gained some weight and my body had a ton of inflammation. On top of this, I juggled school, multiple jobs, and many other commitments I piled onto my plate. I had never been taught about self-care so I continued to focus on my achievements, and disregarded my declining health. I gave all my time and energy to excelling in my work, in my friendships, and in anything that made me feel worthy. On the outside, it seemed like I succeeded in everything I did and I constantly received praise. On the inside, I was suffering. I was living off drive-thrus, venti coffees, and hardly any sleep. Eventually, it all caught up to me.

When I was supposed to be enjoying my freshman year of college, I was diagnosed with an autoimmune disease. I was the sickest I had ever been. I was constantly on antibiotics, had no energy, and would take multiple naps a day. I couldn't focus on school and found college to be extremely difficult. Every aspect of my life suffered. I had no knowledge in natural medicine or healthy eating. Though I was constantly sick, I didn't know how to help myself other than continuing to go back to the doctor and take one prescription medication after another.

The call that saved my health

During this season, my mom was also diagnosed with the same autoimmune disease and we found ourselves looking for answers together. One day, my mom called and said she had went to a health seminar about our condition and learned how we can heal our bodies naturally! I had been feeling so worn out that I would have been willing to try absolutely anything to feel normal again. We quickly made an appointment to see an integrative health doctor to get further testing done and see what holistic treatment would look like for us.

I had never heard of a natural health doctor before, nor had I heard of treating an illness with food and herbal supplements. It was a totally new language for me! I remember meeting with the doctor for the first time and my mind was completely blown. He told me that I could reverse my disease, get off medication, and go back to my normal self if I stuck to his protocol by changing my diet, routines, and everything about my current lifestyle. I was so desperate to feel better; I agreed to do whatever it took to feel well again.

The first thing I did to combat my condition was completely change my diet and daily lifestyle. I gave up caffeine, gluten, dairy, soy, corn, sugar, inflammatory foods, and more. I learned how to cook for the first time, began taking supplements, and created a strict routine that I stuck to. I did everything I could to cut out excess stress in my life, including quitting my corporate job and taking up nannying so I would have less pressure in the workplace.

I learned for the first time that it was okay, and even crucial, to say no to social obligations that wouldn't fit into my new lifestyle.

Let me preface this by saying that this was before wellness, self-care, and gluten-free were household names. No one I knew ate gluten-free and I was often met with negativity from friends and family. Some people thought I was drastically changing my lifestyle to get attention. Since I was never taught to take care of myself, many family members of mine thought I was spending too much time on myself and becoming self-centered. I had been a people pleaser my entire life. For the first time, I was learning that I needed to take care of myself, even if it meant that I would disappoint others. This was a tough reality to face for a young nineteen year old.

It didn't take long before I started feeling better. Within three weeks of living this new lifestyle, my energy started to come back. I began to sleep better, look better, and think better. My constant sinus infections went away and I was able to go a full day without napping. I truly felt like I was experiencing a miracle! I lived an extremely strict lifestyle under a natural doctor's care for a full year after my diagnoses. By the end of the year, I was able to lower the dosage of my medication and live a somewhat normal life. Even though I couldn't eat like all my peers, I didn't mind! I would go to parties in college and sip on water and bring my own carrot sticks to snack on. It may sound crazy, but I was completely content. Nothing in the world could keep me from this new-found healthy lifestyle and wellness mindset because it was healing me from the inside out!

After focusing on healing my health for a year, it was time to heal my soul. I began reading personal development books and spent most of my free time reflecting, processing, journaling, and healing from the negative paradigms I was so accustomed to. I began to prioritize my mental health as well and spent time doing things that infused my life with joy. I distanced myself from toxic relationships and I let go of the never-ending guilt I carried from feeling like I was never good enough. I let God heal my heart in the places it was broken. I was devoted to becoming the woman that God wanted me to be, not who my friends wanted me to be or who my family pushed me to be. I felt convicted to run after self-love and acceptance for myself. I learned how mental health affects physical health and so I was determined to be the best version of myself, not for others, but for me.

Since the culture I grew up in focused on putting down our own needs and desires for the sake of others, I knew that I was not diving into a popular lifestyle. I grew up thinking that in order to be a "good Christian girl" I needed to live a life in complete service to others at all times. During this season of my life, though, I knew I needed to focus on myself and my own well-being. I later realized that I can love and serve others best when I have loved and cared for myself first. This may be a foreign concept to you, but I truly believe that embracing self-love will change your life.

Where I am today

Flash forward six years and I still continue to prioritize my health and wellness above all else. I have learned that self-care isn't selfish, it's essential. I share my journey to wellness because I want you to know that it wasn't an easy process. Nothing worthwhile in life comes easy! I am still prioritizing my health each and every day. I am still working on self-love and self-acceptance. There is no destination, wellness is a life-long journey. This book isn't just about my journey, it's about yours too. You can choose right now to embark on your own personal quest to wellness and self-love. It's not about where you have been. It doesn't matter how you were raised or the trials you have faced in your past, you can learn to love and cherish who you are and who you were created to be.

This book contains the tools needed to start your own journey to self-love and acceptance. I will be sharing exactly what has worked for me and I hope it inspires you to do the work needed to authentically love yourself and grow into the best version of the person you are made to be. I am not a psychologist, nutritionist, dietician, or mental health professional— I am just a girl who has done hard work and continues to do work to overcome struggles each and every day. I'm here with you. I'm just a friend sharing what has worked for me.

As you read this book, I want to encourage you to keep a journal handy. Take notes of any emotions that come up as you read. Reflect on your own life and journey. After each chapter, there will be an action item or topic to journal about. I want to encourage you to take the time to process and give yourself space to reflect on your life and your own personal experiences so that you can learn to love the beautiful person you are.

ACTION ITEM: Have you ever found yourself in a place of self-loathing? Where do you think those negative thoughts stem from? What are your goals in reading this self-love guide? What aspects of wellness do you want to focus on in your own life?

Absolutely. I think that my negative thoughts about myself stem from deep insecurities, anxiety, and the need to please others. My goal is to figure out ways that I can truly find freedom from those things. I want to focus on overall physical + mental health (mostly mental).

2 WHO YOU ARE IS ENOUGH

You are uniquely you. There is no one else on the planet that has been given the exact same strengths, weaknesses, and personality traits as you. You are a valuable player and an asset to those around you. In fact, you are so gifted that you can accomplish anything you want in this beautiful life! But, your worth is not defined by your accomplishments or accolades. Your worth is found in who you already are. The amazing, glorious, and beautiful human that you are! Oh, how I wish this is always how we viewed ourselves.

From the moment you were born, you have been shaped into the person you are today. As a child, you may have been given a treat for behaving. In grade school, we are given gold stars for a job well done. In high school, we are told that we must do well on our

SAT's so that we can get into a good college and get a good job because heaven knows that's the key to a successful life. Maybe you were told that you could do anything you put your mind to, but when you had a bright idea to be an artist or a writer, your dreams were shut down because you were told that you need a stable career. Maybe you were pruned to be this version of yourself that isn't truly who you were made to be. This is the situation I found myself in.

I went to college because that's what I was supposed to do. Simple as that. I had no interest in college. I was completely bored out of my mind in most of my classes. Most of my college years were spent dreaming of the days when I was through with college and my life would really begin. I would dream of doing creative work I was proud of. I dreamed of writing books in coffee shops and testing out recipes for a blog I wanted to start. I even decided to start my own business while in school so that I wouldn't have to get a normal nine to five job once I graduated. Even though I knew deep down in my heart that college wasn't for me, I still went. Why? Because my identity was founded on my accomplishments and success. According to my family, if I go to college, I succeed. Therefore, I went to college.

Now, if you are in college right now, I'm not telling you to quit! Looking back, I am so glad that I stuck it out and got my college degree! It showed me that I can do hard things. Getting that piece of paper that I had been told was so important taught me that sometimes you have to do things you don't necessarily like to get to the place you ultimately want to be. Looking back, I realize that sticking through school and getting my degree taught me important lessons on discipline, hard work, and consistency, which are all very important attributes in the work I do today.

I also don't think it's wrong to listen to the advice of your parents. My parents have taught me so much, and in hindsight, I am thankful I persevered and got my degree. The point I'm trying to make is that my internal motives for going to college were wrong. I felt that if I didn't finish college, I wouldn't be worthy of success. I believed that I would be a failure if I didn't check college off the list of to-do's because my identity was in what I did rather than who I was.

While in school, I also worked. A lot. Throughout my whole life, my family would praise me for being such a hard worker, a go-getter, and a natural entrepreneur. I put a lot of pressure on myself to fit that description. I worked way harder than I needed to in college because I felt that if I could be successful in school AND in work then I would gain extra praise. I spent a lot of time in jobs that did not highlight my strengths or propel me forward in my passions because I believed I needed a professional job. I would often take overtime shifts rather than spend a night with my friends because I felt like that is what a successful person would do. My identity was based on the wrong ideals. Maybe yours is too.

Failure

Maybe you have failed and you carry the shame of failing at something you thought you would excel at. There have been countless times in my life where I have failed and that failure gave me the message that I am not good enough.

During college, I got hired at a job that I was extremely passionate about. I'm telling you, this was a dream job. I was so excited for it and I just knew that this could lead to more potential opportunities in my future career. I only worked there for a few months before I got fired. Yep, the overachiever, hard worker, go-getter got fired. I was completely crushed. I felt that if I couldn't succeed at this job, my creative dream job, how would I ever be able to succeed at having my own business? I learned a couple valuable lessons. First, I am not a details person. It is so hard for me to pay attention to small details, and as much as I have tried to change that about myself, I am simply a big-picture person. The second thing I learned through this experience was that just because I wasn't good at one thing, does not mean I won't succeed at other professional dreams I pursue.

Maybe you have failed at something you believed in so deeply and you are wondering if there will ever be an opportunity for redemption. Let me tell you, it's time for you to create your opportunity for redemption! It's time for you to begin again. You may fail again. You may fail one hundred more times until you get it right, but don't for one second believe that your failures make you any less worthy of success. Remember, your worth is not based on your success, or lack of. You are worthy because you are a human being created for a purpose. Simple as that.

You are loved because you are breathing

When my husband Danny and I were dating, I oftentimes

dealt with doubt and insecurity. Sometimes, I would let those fears get the best of me and I would lash out in anger or instigate a fight. I will never forget one of those nights when I was feeling completely unworthy of love and insecure in my ability to juggle it all: school, work, and being a good girlfriend. I will never forget what Danny said to me, "You are loved because you are breathing." He said it so sincerely that it touched my heart in a new way. I began to cry because I truly couldn't wrap my head around it. Of course I am breathing, I thought. How does that make me loveable? In the past, I had fought to earn love and adoration like it was something I could achieve or win a prize in. Until that point, I had never once believed that I would be loved just because I was me. I was breathing.

Whatever external pressure is telling you who you need to be, don't listen to it. Whatever failure that might be holding you back is nothing compared to the amazing qualities you have simply because you are alive. You are breathing.

We have all been told who we are supposed to be or what we should accomplish at one time or another. Maybe a specific person has put added pressure on you or maybe you put it on yourself. I want to give you permission to give yourself a clean slate. Don't listen to the noise. Just be you.

What we DO is not who we ARE. Embracing who we ARE will be the most important part in DOING what we are truly passionate about.

Who ARE you? Are you a good friend? Do you have a generous heart? Do you have strengths in singing, knitting, or playing mini golf? Are you talented at standing on your head? I'm not asking who you want to be or who you are striving to be. I want to know who you are already. What makes you uniquely YOU!

ACTION STEP: Write out 10-15 qualities that make you uniquely you. They can be truly anything! Try not to focus on who others perceive you as. Think of innate talents or qualities that make you unique!

If you are used to negative self-talk, this action item may be hard to do. If you find this challenging, I want you to start writing things about your physical body. Write out: I have two brown eyes, I have long brown hair, I have two arms, etc. It may seem silly but you need to fall in love with who you already are. So if finding unique qualities or talents is hard to think of, start simple.

> I am: energetic, passionate, a people-person, hard working, intelligent, trust worthy, forgiving, I am able to be friends with many types of people, I have a big heart and deeply care for those around me.

3 WHO DO YOU NEED TO FORGIVE?

In the last chapter, we talked about overcoming the pressures put on us from external people or circumstances in our lives. We also reflected on our natural talents and abilities. As you have been processing through this book, maybe unresolved hurt or bitterness has come up. Maybe you are disappointed in ways you have been treated or have treated yourself. Maybe you have forgotten just how amazing you are because someone once told you that you aren't good enough. Maybe you have spoken so negatively to yourself for so many years that your heart and mind is full of self-loathing thoughts. Whatever the case may be, in order to move forward in your journey to self-love, you need to forgive others and most importantly, you need to forgive yourself. You are not your mistakes. Harboring negative emotions and bitterness will keep you from loving and appreciating yourself. It will also keep you from having authentic relationships with others.

On forgiving others

There may be someone in your life that hurt you beyond repair. You could have been mistreated, abused, or hurt in a way that forgiveness seems unattainable. This chapter may be really hard for you to swallow. If you are feeling emotions rise up against someone who really hurt you, I want you to know that it's okay to hurt. It's okay to feel those emotions. There was a time in my life where I felt so incredibly wronged, and since that person did not apologize, I couldn't imagine forgiving them. These emotions harvested a toxic environment that affected my health and well-being. I knew that I could either let these emotions continue to negatively impact my life or I could learn to forgive. I remember spending a full year of my life journaling about forgiving this person. Every day I would pray and write out my emotions. I would write "I forgive you" over and over even though that was the last thing on earth I wanted to do. I knew that in order to live a life of peace and wholeness, I needed to let it go.

Forgiving someone who does not deserve it does not mean you are letting them off the hook. It doesn't mean that you are forgetting about how you were wronged. It is simply the act of consciously letting go negative emotions that keep you from being the person you were created to be. Resentment is like a brick that we carry through life. It makes everything harder. It keeps us burdened so we can't take on other loads that would better suit our time and interests. It keeps us from being ourselves. If this is an area you really struggle in, I would encourage you to seek professional help. I have gotten professional counseling many times throughout my life and it has been invaluable to my personal growth and development.

On forgiving yourself

I believe that one of the biggest hurdles when it comes to women loving themselves is the negative thoughts they feed into their own minds. Have you ever had a negative thought? Have you ever looked into the mirror and thought unkind comments about yourself? Are you too hard on yourself? Do you spend time criticizing your every word or action? The self-talk that runs through our minds on a daily basis has a huge impact on the person we become. Would you talk to someone else like you talk to yourself? How can you ever love and accept yourself if you don't even like yourself?

If you carry any regrets or failures from your past, it's time to forgive yourself. We are all human and we all make mistakes. We are allowed to mess up, but we must learn to forgive ourselves in order to move past our failures. Harboring shame or regret is only going to keep you from the person you are meant to be!

It's time to forgive

If you have held onto negative emotions towards yourself or someone else, I want to encourage you to let them go. It won't be easy, but I promise that when you can show love and forgiveness to yourself and others, you will begin to see things with more clarity and perspective.

ACTION STEP: Spend some time journaling about forgiveness and any emotions or memories that come up. Write out any person that comes to mind when you think of forgiveness and all the emotions that may come with it. I also want you to write about any past mistakes or failures that you have been carrying with you. After you have put all of this on paper, write out "I let this go." Write this out as many times as you need for as many days or weeks or years that is required. It can take years to fully feel true forgiveness come into your heart for someone who has really hurt you. This isn't a check-it-off-the-list type of step. It can take a long time for pain to heal, and like I said earlier, many times professional help is needed. I am just sharing what worked for me in a season of life where I was carrying a heavy-load of bitterness and self-loathing.

When you write out the things that you need to forgive yourself for, allow yourself to truly let it go. Let the weight of regret slip off of your shoulders. It's not needed anymore. Say this affirmation out loud for as long as it takes until it feels real.

Every day I have the chance to begin again
I am not my mistakes, I am worthy just as I am
I learn more and more each day to be the person I was created to be
I will overcome every hardship that comes my way with grace and integrity

mistakes {
High school 101. Sam .. Nick.
Putting my worth in what boys
said about me. Punishing myself
for the way my body looks (not
eating, taking pills, etc). Drinking to
numb pain.
}

I let this go. I let this go. I let this go.
I let this go. I let this go. I let this go!

4 WHAT MAKES YOU COME ALIVE?

As you begin to let go of the negative parts of your past, the future gets brighter! When we let go of the things that hold us back, we are able to see all the opportunities in front of us much more clearly. One of the biggest things I have learned about finding purpose in life is that we must make time to do the things we love. I have talked to countless people who aren't satisfied with their lives, yet they aren't doing anything to change their circumstances. How are we supposed to love and appreciate ourselves when we don't love or appreciate what we do and how we spend our time?

If you are at a place where you don't truly love yourself, maybe it's time to spend some time doing the things you love! I have learned more about myself and have been the most inspired when I consciously make the time to do things I love. A few years ago, I had a realization that truly changed the trajectory of where I was headed in life. I decided that I was going to pursue the things in life that made me come alive. Doing what makes you come alive are the activities, past-times, or passions that you could do for hours and not know how much time has passed. It could be an activity you've loved since you were a child or the feeling that comes after discussing a new project you are so excited for you can't even sleep.

What are the things that truly make you light up inside? It doesn't have to be something grandeur; it could be super simple. For me, spending time with my girlfriends does my soul some good. I love being a friend and being known by good friends. Five years ago, I had no idea I could turn my passion for authentic relationships into a career, but somehow, by following my passion that is what happened! The entire foundation of my career is simply being a friend and inspiring others. I truly don't think I would have ever found myself in this place if I didn't carve out the time to do what made me come alive.

What else makes me come alive? Going on solo adventures, trying out new coffee shops, and reading a good novel. Part of loving yourself means carving out time for the things you love. You must value yourself enough to do the things that feed your soul. When you do the things that you love, you feel inspired. When you do the things that make you come alive, you will find yourself in a place of gratitude for your life. Gratitude truly will set you free.

Maybe this all sounds foreign because you are so used to living your life based on someone else's approval or expectations for you.

I want to give you permission to believe that you are worthy of doing what you love. Maybe your life is caught up in expectation. The expectations you put on yourself hold you back from doing what your soul truly wants. Maybe you have grown accustomed to pushing down your own wants and desires because of fear, shame, or insecurity. Well friend, we aren't living like that anymore! I believe in more for you.

I'm not talking about living a life of selfishness. Loving yourself and pursuing what you are passionate about isn't selfish. I actually think it is the most selfless thing you can do. Hear me out. There have been different seasons in my life where I was more focused on what I felt I should be doing rather than what I wanted to be doing. This led me down a path of discontentment, anxiety, and self-pity. Let me tell you, there is nothing more selfish than feeling sorry for yourself when you could be choosing to live a life you are passionate about. When I am living in a place of people pleasing, I find that in actuality I do the opposite. My relationships suffer, my business suffers, and my soul suffers when I choose to live the life someone else has for me. It is only when I consciously decided to follow my intuition and pursue the things that made me come alive that I found I had the greatest impact of service to others. Oftentimes, the things that bring us joy and make us come alive lead us to our purpose in life. If you aren't carving out time to do what you love, you could be missing out on the unique ways you were created to change the world!

So, what makes you come alive? What are the things that you wish you could spend more time doing? It's time to reflect and make a list of everything that makes you feel AMAZING. We are so wired to think about what we should do rather than what we want to do, and so this may be challenging. For me, it was almost impossible. Still, as I write this, it's hard for me to decipher what activities bring me the most joy because I'm so wired to be productive all the time.

ACTION STEP: I've learned to experience joy when I cross things off my to-do list. This is not true life-giving joy. True joy is found in the simple moments of pure bliss. What brings you pure bliss? Take some time to journal and write out anything that comes to mind. Try not to let your logical side kick in. For example, treating myself to a spa day gives me pure bliss. That being said, it is not practical for me to live my life at the spa. This list isn't about practicality. We can learn how to practically add in things that bring joy into your life in the next chapter. This is about deciphering WHAT MAKES YOU COME ALIVE! It may not always be practical or logical and that's okay.

Here are a couple of personal examples of things that bring me joy and make me come alive: a spa day with my girlfriends, playing the guitar, taking an afternoon to read a new issue of Magnolia Journal, traveling to new places, trying out new coffee shops, playing board games, being at the lake house with my family, eating sushi, taking photos and being caught in the creative process, picking out a bouquet of fresh flowers, burning my favorite candle, slumber parties, playing in the waves at the beach, getting caught up in a novel, creating a new playlist on spotify, and so much more…

Note: These aren't very extravagant activities. Most of the

items on this list are free and aren't very time-consuming. Your list may look VERY different than mine and that is okay! Just write out the first things that come to mind.

Hiking, playing sports, spending time in the sun with friends, reading, cozy days w/ roomie, anthro candles, naps, playing card games w/ friends, going to the movies w/ mom, self-care nights, working out, traveling, taking pictures, going to the lake

5 LEARN TO SAY NO

Maybe you are reading this and wondering how on earth you will find time in the day to do what makes you come alive. We can make all the excuses in the world on why we won't make time to do something and saying that you are 'too busy' is the biggest of them all. The truth is, you will make time to do what you value. If you value other people's opinions of how you should spend your time, you will do the things that society has deemed valuable. I would encourage you to assess exactly how you are spending your time. How much TV are you watching? How much time are you spending scrolling social media? How many commitments do you have each week that you do out of obligation but don't bring you joy? If you are finding yourself strapped for time, always stressed, and not living in the present, this is the chapter for you. It's time to say NO.

Before we dive into the idea of saying no, let's combat the myth of not having time to do the things that make you come alive. Even though I have tried to improve over the years, I am no expert in time management. I used to be the girl that complained about not having enough time in my day to cross off my to-do list and do things that make me come alive. Then I read, 168 Hours by Laura Vanderkam. It rocked my world and made me realize that, in fact, I have enough time to do anything I choose to. That's the kicker, we get to choose how we spend our time. Time is not in control of us, we are in control of our time. If you are struggling with finding margin in your day to do the things you love, read that book. It changed my entire viewpoint on time management and I believe it will change yours too.

Okay, back to 'saying no'. You can only say yes to the things that are life-giving if you say no to the things that aren't. Saying no isn't about doing less, it's about creating margin in our lives so we can do more of what actually matters. If you take pride in how much you can accomplish in a day, this may rock your world. If multitasking is your second-nature, it's time to reframe your thinking. This is still something I have to work on each and every day. Writing a book has actually been a huge challenge in this area. Gathering my thoughts to take the time and write something so personal isn't just something I can cross off my daily to-do list. The process of writing has required me to make a margin in my life to just think. I've had to set some other dreams on the back-burner so I can give these words my full attention.

Is there something in your life that deserves your full

attention, but you are so focused on crossing off your to-do's that you have forgotten what's most important? How you spend your time, day after day, eventually turns into a lifetime. In this journey to self-love, it is so important that we get a handle on our schedules. If we fill our schedules with our biggest priorities and the things that bring us joy, we will live in a place of gratitude that will radiate into every aspect of our lives.

ACTION STEP: *The Joy Test* ~ I find that I experience the most gratitude and self-love in my life when I am in control of my schedule, filling it with life-giving activities. Obviously, not everything you do may bring you joy, but if the majority of your schedule is dictated by things you loathe, it's time to make a switch. Over the next week, I want you to write out everything you do during the day from the moment you wake up to the moment you go to bed. Make a list of the mundane things you do every day as well as the unique things that vary day to day. At the end of the week, highlight all of the similar mundane tasks and all of the unique activities in different colors. Circle the activities that brought you joy in the last week. Underline the activities that are joy-drainers. What are the things you absolutely loathe doing but always do each week? Lastly, cross out the time suckers. What are the things you do each week that don't bring you joy, and aren't necessary to your well-being, yet, take up your precious time?

This exercise should give you a good perspective on how you are spending your time. How many circles do you have on your paper? Are you spending time doing things that bring you joy? I want to encourage you to spend at least 15 minutes a day doing something you absolutely love. Can you find 15 minutes a day to do something that makes your soul come alive?

When you can carve out time every single day to do something you love, you are telling yourself that you are worth feeling joyful. For example, I love playing my guitar and writing songs. It's been a passion of mine for as long as I can remember. In recent years, I haven't made it a priority to play the guitar every day. I've deemed it unproductive in my head and therefore I don't often make the time to do it. The crazy thing is, whenever I do make the time to play my guitar, I feel rejuvenated and inspired. I feel alive. When I feel rejuvenated and inspired, I am so much more motivated in all aspects of my life. Whenever I play guitar, my confidence is lifted and I feel so grateful for the experience. If that isn't productive to my life, then I don't know what is!

Your time is sacred. You only have 24 hours in each day and we all know that the days go by quick. If you want to live a life of impact, you must learn how to say no to some things so that you can say yes to the right things. If you can learn to show yourself love in this area by managing your schedule in a way that gives you time to recharge, I know that you will find so much more gratitude and contentment in your life.

6 OVERCOMING INSECURITY

I'm not sure you would be human if you didn't deal with insecurity at one point or another. Insecurity is the place in our life where we feel the most exposed in our self-perceived imperfections. Maybe you are insecure in your job, in a relationship, or in your jeans. What I've realized is that as much as we may try to overcome our own insecurities, they will always come back. I used to try and hide my insecurities or avoid thinking about them. I would put up walls and try my hardest to not think about how insecure I was in a new friendship, in building my business, or in my new bathing suit. Pushing down those emotions never worked.

When you push down emotions because of fear or insecurity, you are walking on a tightrope. At some point, the wind is going to blow and you will fall into a black hole of negative self-talk and self-criticism. Instead of trying to forget or hide our insecurities, what if we embraced them? When we recognize our fears and insecurities they lose power over us.

A very personal example for me would be my struggle with anxiety. I struggle with feeling insecure with any type of change or conflict that occurs in my life because I'm afraid that my anxiety will build and initiate a panic attack. Even though this rarely happens, it is still a constant fear of mine. Thinking about feeling anxious makes me anxious and so I often push my insecurities down and try not to think about them. If I don't think about them though, the overwhelming feeling of uncertainty only gets worse. What I've learned is that I need to embrace my struggle with anxiety. I know that I deal with it and so instead of hiding from it, I must choose to face it head-on. I am learning to not react to my anxiety, but instead, be proactive in learning calming techniques that fight off panic. I may not ever overcome my struggle with anxiety, but I can choose to stop hiding from it and instead challenge it. When you acknowledge a weakness in your life, you have influence over it. It can no longer control how you feel, but you can control how you want to feel about it.

I want to give you a little truth-talk on the myth of insecurity. A lot of times when we struggle with an insecurity, we feel isolated and feel as though no one else is going through what we are. Have you ever said, "If only I had hair like her, I wouldn't be so insecure" or "If only I wasn't awkward in conversations then I would have more friends." Let me debunk this for you, you are not alone. Every single person deals with insecurity. Every person on this planet doubts themselves and their abilities, looks, or talents at some point or another. You are not alone. We may all deal with different types of insecurity, but we all deal with it in some way or another.

Body love

Oftentimes, when people think of self-love, they refer to their physical appearance. I believe that there is so much more that goes into self-love then how you look, but I do think it's important to talk about! Loving who you were created to be begins with the heart, but you must also learn to love how you were created to look.

From a young age, we are subconsciously taught how we should look by having outside influences flood our minds. I remember watching music videos on VH1 as a child and seeing singers like Britney Spears and Christina Aguilera wearing next to nothing in regards to their outfit choices. Not only were they wearing barely any clothing, but their bodies were edited to perfection in every way. As I continued to grow up, my mind was constantly infiltrated with what society deemed attractive and how I was supposed to fit into that mold.

As I mentioned at the beginning of this book, I started comparing my appearance with others at a very young age. It wasn't that I hated the way I looked, I just constantly compare myself with others. Since I had a round belly as a child (what child doesn't?), I always compared my stomach with others. I remember being in gymnastics and wearing the same leotard as my team, but as we looked in the mirror and practiced, I would compare how "fat" I was in comparison to my teammates. It seems so silly now since I was probably about 10 or 11 years old at the time, and as a gymnast who practiced 10 hours a week, it was probably impossible for me to gain weight even if I tried!

That's the problem with insecurities. Oftentimes, insecurities are stemmed from lies we tell ourselves or have believed from our childhood. Since I didn't look like my cousin at five years old, I believed the lie that something must have been wrong with me. The lie I believed followed me into adulthood and I constantly felt insecure about my stomach even though there was nothing wrong with it. Eventually, I got so sick that my stomach actually did bulge out because I was dealing with extreme bloat and food sensitivities. When I got sick, I realized that I needed to heal my body from the inside out. To this day, I believe that my constant ridicule and critical thoughts towards my body contributed to me getting sick. It wasn't until I started focusing on my inward health, that I began to appreciate my body and how I looked on the outside. It actually took me going through that hard time with my health to realize that if I'm living a healthy lifestyle, my body starts to look better and my confidence soars.

Think about it, when your body is healthy on the inside, it shows on the outside. If I'm feeding my body healthy and nutrient dense food as well a living an active lifestyle, my body shows it. As I learned to heal my body from its ailments naturally, I began to worry about how I felt instead of how I looked. This mindset shift has healed me from years of believing the lie that I would always keep extra weight on or not be as skinny as I want to be. I have learned to love the body I have been given. Being confident in your body goes so much deeper than your physical appearance. I hope that as you continue to learn to love yourself in other areas, you will grow more confident in the body you were given and how amazing it really is.

I know that this topic can be very sensitive and my experience with body-love may be entirely different than yours. No matter where you are on your journey to body-love, I want to encourage you that as you learn to love yourself in other areas, you will begin to appreciate the amazing and capable body you have been given.

Action Step: *Dry Body Brushing & Oil Massage* ~ Learning to love your body may take a lifetime, but it's time to start treating our bodies with love and respect now. Taking care of your body can look like many different things, but I am going to share a practice I do before I shower that has helped me to nurture and appreciate the body I have.

My secret to glowing skin? Dry brushing. Dry body brushing is actually an ancient form of self-care that has been used in almost every ancient civilization. This form of self-care is said to protect the skin, aid the lymphatic system, and remove dead skin cells. Since I have been dry brushing, my skin has been more soft, smooth, and I have had less clogged pores on my arms and back.

How to:
-Get a wooden body brush that you will only use for dry brushing (not intended to get wet). I order mine off Amazon and get a new one about every 6 months since they are pretty inexpensive.

-Before a shower, spend 5 intentional minutes exfoliating your skin by dry brushing. Brush in a downward motion and use repetitive strokes on the entire body. I dry brush my arms, legs, torso, feet, and back.

-While you are dry brushing, use this as an intentional time to show love for your body. If a critical thought comes into your head, quickly replace it with a positive thought. Do not let any negativity fill this sacred time of self-care.

-After you finish dry brushing, I would recommend giving yourself an oil massage! The practice of oil massage is an ancient Ayurvedic practice that helps to nourish the body and bring moisture back into it. Body brushing can be a little abrasive at times and so I've found that when I give myself an oil massage after, my skin stays hydrated and soft.

-To give yourself an oil massage, first pick an oil. I use Sesame oil in the fall/winter and coconut oil in the spring/summer. It may sound weird to lather yourself in oil you would otherwise use in cooking, but I promise you, it is so good for your skin! After dry brushing, simply massage oil into the areas you body brushed in. Don't worry about being oily because after massaging the oil in, you will shower and all the excess oil your body doesn't need for moisture will come off!

-Shower like normal and experience truly radiant and glowing skin! Aim to do this practice 2-3 times a week for best results. Use this as your time to appreciate the body you have been given and love and care for it accordingly! You're worth it!

7 SELF TALK

In my journey to self-love, I've learned the power our self-talk has on our physical and mental health. What we think is truly what we become. I grew up in an environment where critiques were given more than compliments and so from a very young age, I learned to be very critical of myself. As a child, I learned to be a busybody that rarely rested because my worth was put in what I did, rather than who I was. My critical thoughts would badger me all day long and tell me what I was doing wrong and how I could always be better. I have let negative self-talk invade my mind since I was a little girl, and I'm sure you have too. Negative self-talk is probably the biggest dream-stealer of them all and it makes it almost impossible to experience self-love.

Take an inventory of the thoughts that go in and out of your mind on any given day. Are your thoughts affirming, supportive, and life-giving? Or are they cynical, fearful, and guilt-provoking? Do you speak to yourself like you would speak to your best friend or your worst enemy? Getting a handle on your self-talk is so critical to your growth as a person. Negative self-talk is going to knock you down every time you get back up. It's time to take control of our thoughts.

The three tools I share below are the actions I personally took in order to retrain my brain to encourage positive self-talk and a positive mindset.

Tools to tackle negative self-talk:
- Acknowledging the lies you tell yourself
- Affirming the truth
- Gratitude Practice

Acknowledging the lies you tell yourself:

I believe that taking some time to reflect on how you speak to yourself will be very insightful for you. Instead of going through the motions, I want you to intentionally spend time listening to your thoughts and what they are telling you. Every time a negative or critical thought comes into your head, write it down. This may seem counterintuitive, but it is so important that you acknowledge the lies taking up space in your brain on a daily basis. By writing these 'lies' down, you may realize that you talk to yourself like your worst enemy, not your best friend. As soon as you write down the lie, though, it will lose its power as we begin to focus on the truth.

Here are some examples of critical thoughts I have noticed

swirling around in my head: "You're such a time waster. You've gained weight because you're lazy about going to the gym. You aren't a good friend."

Affirming the truth:

After you have a list of "lies", it's time to affirm the truth! We are all human and we all fall short and make mistakes. This exercise isn't supposed to brainwash us into believing we are a perfect human being. The point of this exercise is to learn to speak to ourselves in a loving way so we can avoid ridiculing our every imperfection. Next to each lie on your list, write out a positive affirmation that confirms the truth about who you are and who you are becoming!

My examples:

LIE: I'm a time-waster
TRUTH: I am learning to manage my time in a way that allows me to balance my time between work, play, and rest. I may not always get it perfect but I am improving every day.

LIE: I gain weight because I am lazy
TRUTH: Weight is not an indication of health. My weight may fluctuate but I aim to live an active lifestyle. Sometimes I need to rest and that does not mean I am lazy. I am smart for listening to my body.

LIE: I am not a good friend

TRUTH: I am a loyal friend that genuinely cares deeply about everyone in my life. I try the best I can to balance being a business owner, devoted wife, and caring friend. There is no such thing as perfect balance, but I aim to do the very best I can.

At first, this may seem very awkward to write about. That's okay if it is. When writing out your "truths", you are affirming the person you aim to be. You are debunking a lie that limits your potential and you are proclaiming the truth that you are more than you give yourself credit for. Please note that there are many times I fall off the bandwagon with my gym routine and I get so busy I forget to call a friend. That does not negate the truth of my intentions though.

What we think, we become. I would rather choose to proclaim affirmations over my life than lies of ridicule that will only tear me down. Since I have implemented this self-care practice into my life, I have found that I am more motivated to go to the gym, call a friend, or use my time wisely because I'm proclaiming those truths over my life. This practice is a powerful one and I hope it radically changes your life like it has mine!

Gratitude Practice:

When I first learned about gratitude practice, I didn't quite understand what it meant and I was also much more cynical than I am now. Adding a practice of gratitude into your everyday self-care routine is crucial because it can actually change your brain chemistry! Like I said before, what you think, you become. If you are filling your mind with thoughts of gratitude, you will naturally become a more joyful, grateful person.

Let's put this into practice...

Let's start with our lies. Turn your lies into thoughts of gratitude.

Here's an example:

LIE: I'm a time-waster
Gratitude thought: I am grateful that I have the opportunity to spend my time doing what I deem valuable.

LIE: I gain weight because I am lazy
Gratitude Thought: I am so grateful that I have a healthy body that's full of energy and allows me to workout but also allows me to rest when I need it.

LIE: I am not a good friend
Gratitude Thought: I am so grateful that I have authentic friendships in my life.

Start with your lies and then move on to other areas of gratitude. Start a running list of everything you are grateful for in your life. Your list doesn't need to be anything profound. Being grateful for a sunny day, a cup of coffee, the birds chirping, and a good yoga class are all very valid reasons to be grateful. Start writing little things you are grateful for and I'm sure your list will be full in no time.

I want to challenge you to begin each day with a list of five things you are grateful for. Over time, I bet that you will begin to have a more positive outlook on your life. This practice is simple, but the results are profound. Don't ever underestimate what the intentional act of gratitude can do for your life!

8 YOUR HEALTHIEST SELF IS YOUR MOST CONFIDENT SELF

I think it's safe to assume that I believe that health and wellness should be a priority in everyone's lives. I've seen first-hand how health can make or break a person's confidence and how optimal health fuels you to dream and achieve more in your life. Even though 'wellness' is a popular phrase nowadays, there is nothing trendy about living a healthy lifestyle. When you are energized, full of vitality, and free from illness, you are able to do the things that make you come alive. When you feel healthy, you naturally feel more confident in all areas because your mind, body, and soul are all in balance. I had to learn the hard way that health is never something to be taken for granted. I am thankful for my health each and every day and I work hard to maintain my health at all costs.

When I talk about health and wellness, I'm not only talking about physical health. Wellness is the trifecta of body, mind, and soul all being in balance. It takes effort to maintain optimal health and it's something that's worth investing your time into. When you invest into your health and wellness, you are creating a better version of yourself that not only benefits you but also benefits everyone around you. It's time to take off the busy badge and intentionally focus on becoming your healthiest self. This is such an integral part of self-care and my hope is that this book inspires you to look at wellness in a new light that doesn't deem it as selfish or indulgent, but as something crucial and life-giving.

Now don't be thinking you don't have the time to focus on wellness. Like I said before, we have time for what we value. Do you value being energized and full-of-life for your family and loved ones? Do you value living a long and healthy life that isn't dictated by stress and sugar? Okay, here we go...

There are three areas of wellness that I believe are super important to focus on; nourishing the body, moving the body, and fueling the mind.

Nourishing the body

Have you ever heard of the phrase 'you are what you eat'? This could not be more true. With every meal you eat, you are fueling your body either in a positive or negative way. The food you consume is absorbed into the body and the nutrients are used as fuel to make all of your systems and organs run properly. I truly believe that one of the most important ways we can practice self-love is by fueling our bodies with nutrient-dense foods that will nourish our bodies and keep us healthy. Eating healthy may not come naturally to you, it certainly didn't to me, but it is worth the effort it takes to re-frame your mindset so that you can show love and respect for yourself in this area. We are given one body and it's our job to treat it with the utmost respect. Your body is truly a temple that is worth taking care of!

I remember the first few months after my scary health diagnosis when I had to completely change my lifestyle and how I ate. I was working at Starbucks at the time and I had to give up all caffeine, sugar, and grains. In case you don't frequent Starbucks often, they pretty much only offer caffeine, sugar, and processed grains. Every single day for the first month of changing my eating habits was a struggle for me. I not only mentally craved a coffee or pastry, but my body did too. I had major headaches and bloating as my body was, quite literally, detoxing all of the unhealthy food I used to eat. It took over a month for me to start to reap the benefits of fueling my body well. I am so glad I pushed through because once I learned what true health and energy felt like, there was no going back for me.

I am not a dietician or nutritionist and so I can't tell you exactly what you should be eating or not eating. I can tell you though, that eating real, unprocessed foods is the best thing you can do for your physical health. Eating a nutrient-dense diet looks like a lot of vegetables, whole grains, and lean meats. Some people process grains better than others just like some people metabolize sugar better than others. It is super important to listen to your body and recognize how you feel after you eat a meal. After each meal, ask yourself this question, "how does my body feel?" Do you feel lethargic and bloated or do you feel energized and content? Eating until you hit a food coma is not eating for wellness. Instead of eating based on emotions or cravings, focus on eating foods that are nutrient-dense and going to help your body run optimally. When you change your mindset on how you consume food, your whole life will improve for the better because you will feel more confident, balanced, and energized!

Moving your body

On my journey to regaining health, exercise was the last habit I picked up. I had always been an active child and did dance and gymnastics throughout my childhood. That changed in high school, though, since I didn't play any traditional sports. Consequently, when I stopped dancing, I unintentionally stopped exercising. I gradually went from a very active teenager to someone who rarely ever worked out. I knew I should exercise and I even had a gym membership, but I was always full of excuses on why I couldn't make it to the gym. I had always figured that the only reason people exercise is to lose weight. I was so uneducated on the benefits of working out for overall health and wellness. When I got sick, I was actually told not to exercise because my body was in a state of extreme stress. After I got my health under control, I knew that I needed to start implementing fitness back into my routine.

Slowly but surely, I began to add workouts into my routine and I realized that working out and eating clean is such a powerful duo to overall wellness!

Just like diet, I've learned that fitness is personal to each individual. Some people feel their best when they run long distances while others are better off with yoga and pilates. It is so important to know your body type and do the types of workouts that are best for you. Each person is different and what works for one person may aggravate your body or leave you exhausted and depleted. Exercise should be something we enjoy and look forward to. If you haven't found a way to exercise that brings you joy, keep looking!

On my exercise journey, I have tried it all. I've spent money on expensive spin classes, yoga studios, pilates and kickboxing. You name it, I've done it. None of these activities were sustainable for me because I would always get bored and could easily talk myself out of going to classes. It wasn't until I found cross-training that I realized I could mix a little bit of everything to form the perfect workout suitable for me. Personally, I love mixing strength training, cardio, and yoga into my fitness routine. I'm also not rigid in my routine. I listen to my body at all times. If I'm feeling particularly exhausted one day, I won't go to the gym and I don't feel bad about it. Some days my exercise simply consists of a long walk. I think it's important to view fitness as living an active lifestyle, not making sure you schedule in a certain number of workouts each week. When you view fitness as a way of loving yourself and self-care, it becomes less about the type of exercise or how many calories you burn, and more about how you feel emotionally and physically.

When you treat your body with the utmost respect by choosing to eat nutritious foods and exercising regularly, you will begin to feel more confident in who you are and who you were created to be. When you make your health a priority, you are showing yourself love in such an important way. Choosing to invest into your health each and every day is going to pay off for years and years to come.

Fuel your mind

Eating nutritious foods and living an active lifestyle are two key elements of good health, but there is also a third component that I've learned is equally as important. Mental health is such a crucial part of overall wellness. What we think is truly what we become. I believe that if our minds are inundated with negative and critical thoughts about ourselves, it will eventually impact our physical health. Just like we need to eat healthy foods and live an active lifestyle to have a healthy physical body, we need to intentionally focus on making sure we have optimal mental health as well. It's the third part of the health trifecta and it's worth investing in.

For years, I focused on regaining health in my physical body but never prioritized my mental health. I lived a busy life of go-go-go and never gave myself time to think about how I was doing emotionally. I had the mindset that I could power through any hardship I faced without thinking about the impact that it had on my mental health. In our society, especially as a woman, I feel as though there is an expectation we put on ourselves that we are supposed to 'do it all' effortlessly and without complaint. We also live in a day and age where everyone's highlight reel is plastered for all to see and that can leave us comparing ourselves and thinking negative thoughts about our own lives. Like I said before, what we think is what we become. It's our job to fuel our mind with positive influences so that we can focus on the good and have the mental capacity to do what we are called to do in this beautiful life we live.

Diving into personal development

One of the most powerful tools I have utilized to become the person I want to be is diving into personal development. When you learn to love yourself and who you were created to be, you will want to become the best version of yourself. You are worth investing in! It is only when you fill your cup up each morning with personal development, that you will be able to pour that out to others and serve and love the people in your life.

In this day and age, there are countless resources out there for personal development. There truly is an unlimited amount of information at our fingertips. In my opinion, choosing not to devote time to personal growth is a choice of ignorance. I've been told my whole life, 'if you aren't growing, you're dying.' Spending time to intentionally grow as a person and focus on personal development will trickle positive effects on so many areas of your life! Here's my personal resources for personal development:

Reading

I am constantly reading personal development books. I'm the type of person who reads multiple books at a time and one of them is always a book centered around personal development in some capacity. Here are a few of my all-time favorite personal development books. I'm always updating this list on my website as well on livewellwithlo.com!

Girl Wash Your Face- Rachel Hollis
Big Magic-Elizabeth Gilbert
Present Over Perfect- Shauna Niequist
High Performance Habits- Brendon Burchard
The 7 Habits of Highly Effective People- Stephen R. Covey
168 Hours- Laura Vanderkam

Podcasts

Over the last year, I've dived head first into the podcast world. I listen to a podcast almost every single day and they instantly motivate and inspire me. I listen to all types of podcasts but my favorite podcasts are on health, wellness, business, or personal development. Here are some of my favorites!

The Melissa Ambrosini Show
The Cabral Concept
Rise Podcast
Second Life
The School of Greatness by Lewis Howes

Other Healthy Practices for Mental Health

I wanted to end this section on mental health with sharing my favorite practices for doing less. So often we can cram our days with as much activity or productivity as possible and we forget to just be. Maybe you've got the personal development piece covered but you are still feeling stressed, anxious, and imbalanced emotionally. If that's you, it's time to slow down and intentionally carve out time for rest.

Sleep

Let's talk about sleep. In my opinion, this is probably the cheapest and most effective way to positively affect your mental health. Our society runs by the notion of "I'll sleep when I'm dead." With this mindset, you'll probably be dead sooner than later. Ha. All joking aside, sleep is so critical to mental health!

I'm not a doctor and so I won't list out all of the studies and research that support this claim, but you can Google the benefits of sleep and you will see hundreds of studies supporting this argument. The hours of sleep needed vary from person to person but getting at least eight hours of sleep a night seems to be the sweet spot for most people. If you aren't getting enough sleep or you are constantly exhausted and running off of ample amounts of caffeine, it's time to start prioritizing rest into your self-care practice. Saying yes to sleep may mean saying no to a coffee date or a workout class or even your work. It all comes back to values.

Your health, wellness, and mental state are worth the sacrifice it takes to keep you rested. You could be eating healthy, working out, and reading all the books in the world, but if you aren't sleeping, your body will begin to break down fast.

Journaling

This is a self-care practice that I have been doing my whole life. Journaling is one of the most therapeutic practices for me because it relieves my mind from carrying the little stressors of everyday life. When my thoughts feel cluttered and anxiety begins to creep in, I take out my leather journal and write everything down.

If you aren't used to journaling, it may take some time, especially if you aren't used to authentically expressing your feelings or emotions. Carve out some space during your day to jot down any thoughts, feelings, or emotions that come up. I like to make journaling a sacred practice by lighting a candle, putting on my favorite playlist, and making a cup of tea. Write about what you are going through in life and everything that's on your plate. Write out anything you can think of that could be bringing you stress and let it all out on the paper. You don't have to just write about the hard stuff either. Write out your victories, what makes you laugh, and all the things you are thankful for! I have noticed that I feel more connected to myself emotionally and more aware of my mental health when I spend intentional time journaling every day.

Meditation

Okay, I've got to be honest, it's hard for me to consistently practice meditation, even though I know that the benefits are boundless! Learning to add meditation into your daily practice isn't for the faint of heart. If you are anything like me, the thought of sitting still for an extended period of time with the sole purpose of thinking about nothing sounds like torture. I've been there. I feel you. We'll get through this together. Because you see, implementing a meditation practice into our daily routines is one of the best things we can do for our mental health. The act of meditation in and of itself calms the mind, eases nerves, and brings you back to the present. During the seasons where I am practicing daily meditation, I feel centered and grounded and am able to cope better with stress.

I completed yoga teacher training two summers ago, which taught me the extensive benefits of meditation. Learning to meditate was hard, even torturous at times, but it brought me so much clarity and peace. My favorite type of meditation is guided meditation because you have someone leading you through it. I have used numerous resources and apps for meditation and I think they are all great! Download an app like Calm or Headspace and commit to meditating every day for a month. You don't have to sit in silence for an hour, just give yourself five or ten minutes! When it gets hard, and it will, don't quit. It is so important that you give yourself intentional time each and every day to just be still. If you are the praying type, like me, the Bible says to "be still and know that I am God." When you allow yourself to give up control, and be still in your own life, you can surrender your fears, anxieties, and stressors to a power greater than your own.

These are the tools I have used to fuel my mind and train my mindset to be a place of gratitude and positivity. I hope that you choose to add some of these tools to your own toolbox to transform your mindset, which will change your life! Keeping your body, mind, and soul in balance is so crucial for experiencing self-love and overall wellness. Even if you have been ingrained with the thinking that you are not worth spending all this effort on, let me reiterate that you are, indeed, worth the effort. You were created to do incredible things and lead an incredible life with passion and purpose! It is your job to take the steps necessary to make sure that you are living and serving with a full cup. Put your oxygen mask on first, friend.

9 TAKE THE ROAD LESS TRAVELED

I am fully aware that many of the topics I talk about in this book are counter-cultural. If I didn't learn this stuff growing up, I'm pretty sure you didn't either. It took me years of wrestling with my own thoughts, insecurities, and fears before I came to peace with the idea of self-love. Once I started implementing self-love and wellness into my daily life, my life changed so drastically that I knew I'd never be able to go back to my old way of living. You see, I have never been as healthy, joyful, and fulfilled in my entire life. Not only that, I also feel like I am able to give so much of my time and energy in service of others because I'm coming from a place of peace and balance rather than un-ending stress and people pleasing.

Throughout my journey, I've had my fair share of naysayers

and people who have watched from the sidelines, observing this new lifestyle, but never embarking on it for themselves. Living a life of wellness and radical self-love takes a lot of inner-work. Living a completely authentic life is hard when we live in a society where busyness, people-pleasing, and constant unmet expectations cloud our days. Some days it's hard to live in a mindset of gratefulness when we are spending the precious minutes of our lives scrolling Instagram, watching brainless Netflix shows, or liking our grandma's cat photos on Facebook. Not that any of those things are bad (my guilty pleasure is The Real Housewives) it's just that so many people would rather cloud their days with distractions than do the work necessary to maintain optimal emotional, mental, and physical health.

    Our days make up our lives. I remind myself daily of the simple truth that each moment matters. How I spend my mornings, days, and evenings is how I spend my life. Take an inventory of your last week, if it were your last week here on earth, is that how you would spend it? What would you do differently? I want you to absolutely love your life. I want you to live each day with passion and purpose. I'm tired of seeing so many amazing women waste their potential because they are unwilling to do the hard work it takes to get to the other side. Working through your past, your insecurities, and your fears is hard. Learning to be still and allow your true thoughts and emotions to arise is sometimes scary. Prioritizing your well-being for the first time in your life may mean that you have to say no to other good opportunities or other people's expectations. All of this is worth it. All of this leads to a joy-filled life. When you experience genuine love for who you were created to be, you will experience more joy in your life then you can even imagine. When we push past the unrealistic expectations, the people-pleasing, and the busyness, we create space for a meaningful joy-filled life.

Take the road less traveled and you will see so much more.

Changing the world starts with you

As we come to the end of this journey, I want you to think about your own life and what tangible changes you need to make to live a life of wellness and self-love. I truly believe that if each of us lived our lives with this new mindset, that we would change the world. Imagine a world where people served others out of love and joy, rather than the expectations they put on themselves. Imagine a world where we focused less on how we looked and more on how we felt. Imagine a world where we can give others our full hearts and attention, rather than just our leftovers from a stressful day. I believe that all of this is possible. I believe that if we were to just realize how beautiful and amazing and talented we all are as individuals, that we would use those gifts to change the world. It's time to stop hiding behind the phone, behind the insecurities, behind the busyness, and behind the hurt. It's time to do the inner-work so that you can shine your light on the world, just as you were created to do.

10 AFFIRMATIONS

I wanted to write the last chapter on affirmations because I believe they are a powerful tool you can use to transform your mindset into one of acceptance and self-love. Whenever I am facing insecurities, doubt, or a negative mindset, I oftentimes use affirmations to help remove the lies I tell myself and fill my mind with affirming language. I also think of affirmations as goals we can speak into our lives. For example, I like to speak affirmations of health over my life to reiterate my intention to focus on making healthy choices every day. You may be thinking that this sounds a little 'woo woo' and I want to assure you that there is nothing 'new age' about using affirming language to train your brain to focus on gratitude and joy!

Here are six affirmations that I wrote to help me focus on gratitude and joy in multiple areas of my life. These are six different topics that I have had insecurities in and I'm sure some of you have as well. I challenge you to speak an affirmation to yourself out-loud every morning and just see how amazing it feels when you start each day with a grateful heart.

Self-image affirmation

I was created to be inherently beautiful
Every part of my body makes me who I am
I treasure my body and treat it with utmost care
I nourish my body and always speak of it kindly
Each feature of mine was created to be exquisitely unique
I am blessed to be able to walk, talk, and
share my inner light with the world
I am beautiful and will share my beauty with
the world in love and grace

Health affirmation

I wake up each morning with a breath of fresh new life,
Ready for whatever the day brings my way
My body is brimming with energy and
clarity to do all that needs to be done
My immune system is strong and will fight off any illness
My organs work perfectly and efficiently in all ways
I am capable of so much because my
health is thriving and sustaining
I show my body the love and respect it
deserves every single day so that I will live to be
Strong, vibrant, and full of energy all the days of my life

Confidence affirmation

I can accomplish anything I put my mind to
I am perfectly capable of achieving incredible things
I do my best in all circumstances
I will not diminish or undermine my greatness
There are unique giftings that only I
have that need to be shared with the world
In everything I do, I will rise to the occasion
because I have what it takes to overcome
any obstacle that may come my way
I am confident in who I am and I believe
that the best is yet to come

Affirmation against fear

Fear has no place in my life
I am whole, I am safe, I have everything I need
Even though uncertain circumstances will come,
I will face them with courage
Fear is an emotion that I will face,
But I will not let it control me
When obstacles and various hurdles seem to overwhelm me,
I will hold onto hope that is bigger than myself
Fear has no place in my life,
So I will live my life in joy and gratitude each and every day

Affirmation on purpose

My life is a journey to finding passion and purpose
This journey may take a lifetime but I will
embark on it one step at a time
I don't have it all figured out, I just need to show up to be a
better version of myself each and every day
I was created to accomplish amazing things
My life has more meaning and purpose
that I can even comprehend
I get to live this beautiful life and be on
this journey to find my life's calling
Step-by-step, day by day, I will live each
day with passion and purpose

Affirmation on contentment

I am immensely blessed
I have everything I need
Each day, I choose to live in thankfulness
for all that God has blessed me with
Material wealth and possessions
come and go like the wind
But I will hold no meaning there
The most important parts of my life are the
intangible things I am blessed with every day
Love and joy
Peace and patience
Friendships and loved ones
I am content in everything I am,
and everything I have
I am lacking nothing

In Closing:

Currently, I'm sitting in a hospital room with my sweet friend who unexpectedly suffered a stroke yesterday. Over the last 24 hours I've questioned everything I've ever believed about health and wellness, and I've been affirmed even more about how crucial it is that we take care of ourselves. We often take our health for granted until something tragic hits us or someone we love and we are dealt a huge dose of perspective on what the meaning of life truly is. Life is not about accolades or material possessions or a job well done. Life is about love, relationships, living out our own unique calling, and making an impact. Throughout the process of writing this book, I have been affirmed even more that self-love is not selfish. We have been given this one body, mind, and soul, and it's our job to nurture it to the best of our abilities. It is only when we put our oxygen masks on first, that we can begin to help others.

Throughout these pages, I have poured out my heart and soul in sharing everything I have learned about self-love and living the life you are called to live. I've shared my personal stories and experiences in the hopes that my story will inspire you on your own journey. Living a life of wellness and self-love is a life-long journey and it's up to you to embark on it one step at a time. If you are tired of being tired, it's time to invest into your wellness. If you are tired of negative self-talk, it's time to do the steps necessary to change your mindset. If you are tired of living a life of people-pleasing, it's time to dig deep and figure out what sets your soul on fire so you can do the things that YOU want for your life, not anyone else.

I hope that in this season, you choose to love the amazing person you are. I hope you choose to speak positively to yourself, to let yourself rest, to encourage yourself do the things that make you come alive. I hope and pray that you begin to take your health seriously and take small actions every day to become the best person you can be. I hope you realize as you begin to invest in yourself that you, in turn, have more energy to pour into others. I hope that your acts of self-love begin to trickle down into your family, your friends, and your community. If we want to truly change and impact the world in a meaningful way, it starts with you. It starts with us. Let's do this.

ACKNOWLEDGEMENTS

I am so beyond grateful for the village that has come alongside me to help me put these words to paper and share them with the world. I would not have been able to pull this off without the incredible people in my life giving me wisdom, encouragement, and the gentle nudge to "stop rambling on and on". ha.

Thank you, thank you Makenna Holford, my very first friend on this earth and the best editor I could have asked for. I knew I could trust you with such personal words because you've known me, quite literally, from the beginning.

Thank you to Sarah Leeworthy for being the most incredible sidekick on this journey. Thank you for your patience in listening to my rambles and ever-changing plans and helping me stay focused on my mission. With every new project idea I have, you rise to the challenge to help me bring it to life and I am so so thankful for you.

Thank you Carli Wentworth for everything you do for me. I don't know what I would do without your friendship in my life. You have seen this passion project of mine from start to finish and I am so thankful for your editing advice, cover photography, and all the ways you have helped me pull this together.

Thank you to my tribe. My best friends. You know who you are. Your love and support has given me wings. I love you all.

Thank you to my mama, Leanne Calvert, and precious grandmother, Della Johnson, for all of your edits and advice! I am thankful for the strong women in our family and I am thankful to have been raised by you both.

Thank you to my dad, Papa Fro, for teaching me that hard work is only worth it if you get to enjoy your life in the process. Thank you for reminding me to rest and not take things so seriously.

Thank you to my sweet, sweet husband, Danny, for empowering me in all of my dreams. I love dreaming with you.

& lastly, thank you to YOU. Yes, YOU. Thank you for reading this book. Thank you for trusting me and reading what I have to say about your one and only precious life. I am grateful for your friendship, whether online or in person, I've got your back.

LET'S BE FRIENDS!

Now that you know me pretty well, I would love to get to know YOU! Follow along on Instagram where I post all things health, wellness, and personal growth! **@livewellwithlo**

Ready to start your journey to self-love and wellness? Reset your morning routine with a nutritious smoothie from my FREE E-book *Live Well With Smoothies*. Available for a free download at **livewellwithlo.com**

Want more wellness inspiration tips and inspiration? Follow along on my blog where I post recipes, self-care tips, and weekly motivation.

I can't wait to connect with you further. We're on this wellness journey together!

Live Well,
Lo

REFERENCES

Burchard, B. (2017). High Performance Habits: How extraordinary people become that way. Carlsbad: Hay House.

Covey, S. R. (2016). The 7 Habits of Highly Effective People. San Francisco, CA: Franklin Covey.

Gaines, C., & Gaines, J. (n.d.). Magnolia Journal.

Gilbert, E. (2016). Big Magic: Creative Living Beyond Fear. London: Bloomsbury.

Hollis, R. (2018). Girl, Wash Your Face: Stop believing the lies about who you are so you can become who you were meant to be. Thomas Nelson.

Niequist, S. (2017). Present Over Perfect: Leaving behind frantic for a simpler, more soulful way of living. Thorndike, ME: Center Point Large Print.

Vanderkam, L. (2011). 168 Hours: You have more time than you think. London: Penguin.

Made in the USA
Columbia, SC
15 January 2019